Get Healthier with Whole Raw Asafoetida

A Practical Guide to Live Longer
How to Use, Where to Buy, Substitutes, Health Benefits and Recipes

The information herein is offered for informational purposes solely and is universal as so. The presentation of the information is without contract or any type of guarantee assurance.

The trademarks that are used are without any consent, and the publication of the trademark is without permission or backing by the trademark owner. All trademarks and brands within this book are for clarifying purposes only and are the owned by the owners themselves, not affiliated with this document.

Table of Contents

Introduction

There is a famous saying that states that "You are what you eat." This simply means that the status of your health and physical wellbeing is highly informed by what you ingest into your body day-in-day-out. If you can embrace the habit of eating not just good food but nutritious food and take regular exercise, then you are good to go. Always have it at the back of your mind that not all good foods are nutritious, but all nutritious foods are good foods. This is because what is referred to as good food is subjective and therefore may not be explicitly defined.

This book seeks to educate you about one of the good and nutritious foods out there. The food in question is known as asafoetida. Asafoetida is a food ingredient and supplement. It is also medicine for a plethora of diseases and conditions. That's rather useful to you. These facts are some of the reasons why you should want to learn all about this so-called asafoetida. Fortunately, that is the objective of the book.

- ☐ The first chapter of the book will talk about what asafoetida means, the various names of asafoetida and the derivation of the names, the origin of asafoetida itself, and how to make optimal use of it.
- ☐ The second chapter will inform you about the plethora of health benefits that can be derived from taking or ingesting asafoetida.
- ☐ Almost all things; food or whatever have their substitutes. Therefore, you have to know the alternatives of asafoetida too. This will be outlined in the third chapter.
- ☐ Storage and preservation of food are almost if not equally as important as eating the food, because,

without them, food will decompose and ultimately become useless to you. Chapter four will explain how you can preserve and store asafoetida.

☐ The fifth and last chapter will explain how to cook asafoetida and the trusted recipe to guide you.

Now, back to business!

Chapter 1: What is Asafoetida and How to Use It

Asafoetida, also known as hing, is a medicinal plant that has been available and used since before the time of Alexander the Great. For this reason, we can call it a very ancient plant.

Origin; Asafoetida = aza (Persian) + foetidus (Latin). Aza means mastic or resin, while foetidus means fetid or foul or stinking. From this illustration, it is safe to say that asafoetida is a foul-smelling mastic or resin. Asafoetida can be found in plentiful quantities in countries in the Middle East and Central Asia, especially India and Iran. In some history books, it is even believed to have originated from Europe to the rest of the world, thanks to Alexander's expedition in ancient Persia. Although, it became rare after the fall of the Roman Empire.

Asafoetida has been called many things by many different tribes, races, and cultures. The Hindu tribe call it hing, the Swahili people of Kenya call it mvuje, the Arabs call it haltit, the Spanish call it asafoetida, and Germans call it stinkasant. Other common names for it are; devil's dung and stinking gum which can be attributed to its natural foul odor.

Description; asafoetida plant is cultivated perennially. It belongs to the Apiaceae plant family, just like celery, parsley, and fennel. At maturity, it grows up to approximately two meters (2m) high with hollow stems, yellow flowers, green leaves, and taproots or carrot-like roots. From its stem and root, a resinous structured gum is secreted. This whitish colored resin then dries and hardens into dark amber when exposed to the sun; a flavorsome and plastic-like resin which is scrapped off then crushed into a powdery spice called asafoetida that is used to add flavor to food and also as medicine. In some places, it is blended together with other foods like rice that is used in cooking.

The whole asafoetida plant has a distinctive unpleasant smell; however, it doesn't stay foul forever. Once boiled, the lousy odor dissipates into an onion smell which isn't so bad. In that regard, it is synonymous with locust beans. Fresh locust beans also emit an unpleasant smell but once they are cooked, it loses that attribute.

Composition; asafoetida is made up of resin (40%-60%), volatile oil (10%-20%), ash (2%-10%) and gum (25%). Each component is also made up of sub-components that have a part to play in why asafoetida looks the way it does, smells the way it does, and its nutritional value. The volatile oil component is made up of several organo-sulfide compounds that are rich in sulfur; hence, the unpleasant smell.

How to Use Asafoetida

Asafoetida is an antispasmodic and opiate-like substance that promises swift relief from stomachache (the digestive variety), flatulence from legumes, and colic pain among others. As it was hinted in the introduction of the book, asafoetida can be used as a medicine, as a food ingredient, and much more; therefore, it is essential you know how to use it for each of the purposes already mentioned above to get the best out of it. For proper and efficient use of asafoetida, you have to be conversant with the different forms it naturally assumes and those it can be transformed into.

Forms of Asafoetida

- Water-soluble: The resin expelled by the trunk and root of the asafoetida plant is milky or whitish in color. As long as it is extracted before it is exposed to excess sunlight, it is eligible to be boiled in water which dilutes it down, thereby toning down its potency (a form of processing).
- Oil-soluble: Once the milky colored resin is exposed to air and sunlight for a considerable amount of time, it darkens into a dark amber or reddish-brown color. These transformations occur naturally and increase its potency in the form of smell, flavor, and texture. The dark-colored asafoetida is boiled in hot oil to dilute it, thereby toning down its potency in the process. Boiling it in water will not give satisfactory results.
- Powdered: This form of asafoetida is somewhat processed. Either the white or the reddish-brown colored types are eligible to be grounded into powdered

form. The advantage of this is that it can be easily mixed with other neutral ingredients such as turmeric, wheat flour, rice flour, etc., for cooking purposes.

- Capsule: Asafoetida, in this form, is used for medicinal purposes. It is taken with warm water to take care of the ailments it is being used for. After the freshly scraped resin is boiled in water, or oil as the case may be, it is broken into smaller pieces (pill size), and then stored in airtight containers.

Now, how are these Asafoetida forms used?

Do not forget that the leaves, fruits, shoots, and roots of the asafoetida plant are all useful and can be utilized for one thing or the other.

☐　　**As food**: Asafoetida is used as a spice in cooking to either enhance the original flavor of the food or to add that onion and garlic flavor to the food. In the past, the raw form of asafoetida was grounded with stones or harmers until it became either granulated to powdery, then it was used that way to flavor meat, vegetables, soup, etc. In modern times, the blended raw form is mixed with other food condiments especially rice flour and turmeric.

In India and Iran, especially, it is used in the majority of their traditional dishes. In fact, it is used as an ingredient in the majority of the vegetarian dishes in India, particularly in those places that are not religiously or culturally allowed to add onion or garlic.

Furthermore, the leaves and young shoots of the asafoetida plant are eaten as vegetables, while starch from the roots is used to make porridge.

☐   **As medicine**: Asafoetida is used to cure a lot of ailments in the body. As a medicine, it is used in different parts of the world for various medicinal purposes. Even the leaves and flowers of the plant are not exempted. For instance, in India and Thailand, powdered asafoetida is mixed mix water or alcohol to form a paste which is then applied to the abdomen to aid digestion or treat indigestion. In Brazil, the leaves and trunks are dried and then boiled, which results in a concoction. This concoction is used as an aphrodisiac by the men. The list goes on and on.

Principally, asafoetida as used as a medicine for internal and external purposes. Internally, it is taken as a pill called 'teardrop' to cure ailments or as an enema; an injection made up of five grams of asafoetida boiled in two to three liters of water.

Externally, some people use it directly on the skin and as one of the ingredients in skin-care products to clear calluses and treat skin inflammations, although there is no authentic scientific proof of its effectiveness.

Chapter 2: Health Benefits

The health benefits of asafoetida cannot be overemphasized. Some of these benefits have been passed down from generation to generation since it was discovered. Therefore, the benefits of asafoetida can even be regarded as a cultural phenomenon. The reason for this arises from the fact that different cultures derived particular benefits from the use of asafoetida apart from the general benefits of it. This does not, however, mean that these benefits are not explored by the whole world. As a result of globalization, advancement in science and technology, once a phenomenon has been scientifically proven or there is clear proof from some other means of its effectiveness, it becomes generally accepted as the culture of the whole world. For better understanding, here are some indigenous asafoetida benefits;

- The traditional Chinese people consumed asafoetida to destroy worms or other parasitic organisms inside the body. The anthelmintic properties in asafoetida help to stun or kill these parasites once ingested with little to no harm to the host.
- In Malaysia, the women chew dried asafoetida, and in Nepal, they take water extracts of it as preventive and curative measures of amenorrhea.
- Moroccans take asafoetida to stem convulsions or as an antiepileptic supplement.
- Dried asafoetida (gum) is used in Saudi Arabia to treat several respiratory diseases such as asthma, whooping cough, and bronchitis.

In some other countries, asafoetida is used for some of its other health benefits. The consensus is that asafoetida has multitudinous benefits. In the following points, a number of the different health benefits of asafoetida will be outlined in more detail. It may include those already stated above but, in more details, (the healing process).

- **Pain relief capabilities;**
  Asafoetida has been proven to be an excellent pain reducer or outright eradicator regardless of the intensity of the pain. Pain as a result of earache, toothache, headache, and migraine, to mention a few, are relieved due to the anti-inflammatory, antioxidant properties of asafoetida. Asafoetida reduces the inflammation in the blood vessels in the affected areas thereby, relieving the pain.
  For earache, a paste made from a mixture of hot coconut oil and asafoetida powder which is applied when cooled. Toothache on the hand is relieved by mixing the powder with lemon juice then applying it to the affected area with a ball of cotton wool. Mixing a pinch or two with your food or with a warm glass of water does the job too when ingested.
- **Prevent cardiovascular problems;**

One of the most occurring cardiovascular problems is hypertension, especially in adults, and it is caused by high cholesterol levels and high triglyceride levels. Coumarin (one of the components of asafoetida) prevents blood clotting through vasodilation (dilation of the blood vessel through the relaxation of the wall muscles). This allows blood to flow properly and facilitates blood thinning. All these processes culminate in the lowering of blood pressure and the proper running of the entirety of the cardiovascular system. Vasodilation can be achieved through the ingestion of the water extract asafoetida.

- **Prevents respiratory issues and improves the immune system;**

When mucus and phlegm are in excess in the respiratory tract, they clog it up, thereby causing breathing problems. Asafoetida helps to remove the excesses. Furthermore, it is packed with chemicals such as; umbelliferone, diallyl-sulfide, azulene, diallyl-disulfide, ferulic acid, luteolin, etc., that are responsible for killing disease pathogens and reducing inflammation in the respiratory tract thereby improving the immune system in the process.

For a home remedy, a paste made from water and powdered asafoetida is applied on the chest to take care of minor cough and breathing issues. However, for more severe issues like inflammation of the walls of the airways in the lungs (bronchitis), asthma and whooping cough, asafoetida is used in conjunction with other herbal plants such as ginger, honey, white onion, betel leaf, etc.

- **Blood sugar regulation;**

Asafoetida is an excellent diabetes inhibitor. The combination of ferulic acid and tannins in the extract of asafoetida when introduced into the body help to accelerate the production of insulin in the pancreas, thereby regulating the blood sugar level. Therefore, adding a pinch or two to your food every day or every other day would not hurt but rather help you, especially if you are at high risk of becoming diabetic.

- **Placebo of women maladies;**
There are a lot of issues afflicting women, and it has a lot to do with their reproductive health. Some of the issues include but are not limited to; menstrual cramps, fertility problems, leucorrhoea, and premature labor.

Menstrual cramps are a result of obstruction of blood flow. Therefore, the use of asafoetida helps to relieve the pain since it is a natural blood-thinning agent. Also, asafoetida enhances the discharge of progesterone which culminates into easier blood flow and pain relief.

The anti-bacterial and anti-viral properties of asafoetida also facilitate the rapid treatment of leucorrhoea (you know that yellowish or whitish discharge from the vagina).

Asafoetida's ability to facilitate the enhanced secretion of progesterone helps to prevent issues such as sterility, premature labor, and the likes.

- **Preventive and curative placebo for bowel problems;**
Asafoetida has always been one of the age-old home remedies for bowel problems. Out of all the health benefits of asafoetida, the ones related to the stomach, bowel, gut, etc., go across borders (i.e., it is common to most countries and cultures all over the world)

Bowel issues such as indigestion, intestinal flatulence, diarrhea, bloating, intestinal worms or parasites, and Irritable Bowel Syndrome (IBS) among others can be solved by taking asafoetida in the right way.

Some people have a sensitive stomach so that when they take lentils and other legumes, they are afflicted with excessive intestinal flatulence. Therefore, if you fall under this category, using asafoetida to spice your food when you cook takes care of the problem.

Taking asafoetida fast-tracks digestion which prevents indigestion and bloating. Apart from consuming it through your food, you could simply put a pinch or two in a glass of water, mix well then drink. You will get similar results.

- **Preventive measure for cancer;**
  Regularly ingesting asafoetida helps you to protect your body and the cells in your body from cancerous cells. The rate at which people are susceptible to cancer varies. Some get it from the things they eat, some from chemicals they are regularly exposed to, while others inherit the gene from their parents. Regardless of your susceptibility, regular consumption of asafoetida will be good for you since it is a good anti-cancer and antioxidant agent.

Finally, asafoetida should be taken in moderate quantities because there are severe consequences for overdosing on it. Some of the milder ones are; nausea, diarrhea, and disruption of the menstrual cycle. Too much of it may even lead to the acceleration of the condition you trying to treat.

Wow! Congratulations!

Do you know that **67%** of the readers **don't finish** the book they are reading and that a relevant percentage **don't even start the second chapter**?

You are on the good track to finish this useful practical guide and my family and I congratulate you for this! :)

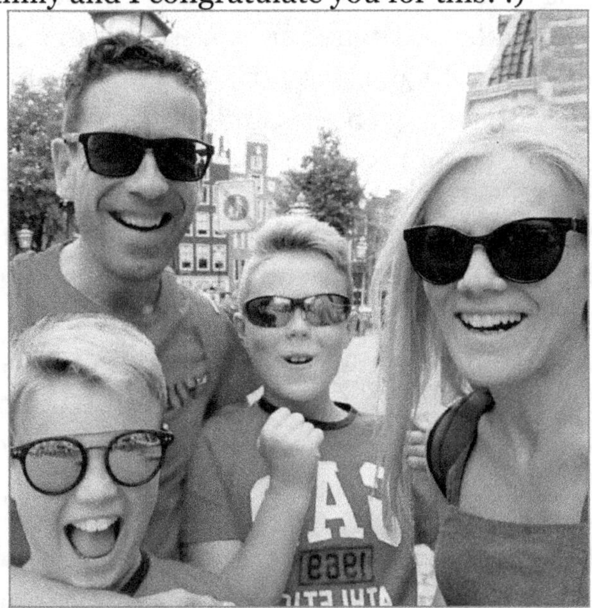

In fact, this book is fully practical with no fluff and I spent many cups of coffee to put it together.

Hope you like it and please leave a review in order to help me as an author and to improve the content of this book.

Your review is very important. I will read it very carefully as it will be used as a tool to refine my work! Thank you!

CLICK HERE TO LEAVE FEEDBACK ON AMAZON
If you're undecided, just leave the review later...

Ah! By the way, this photo was taken last Summer in Amsterdam. Very hot day! :)

Chapter 3: Substitutes for Asafoetida

Almost everything, food, gadgets, drinks, etc., has substitutes these days, and asafoetida is not an exception. When something has a substitute, it means there is something else that has very similar attributes or causes the same effects as it does. Having knowledge of the other available options allows you the luxury of making choices and prevents you from being in situations that cannot be helped.

When it comes to food substitutions, you need a certain level of skill and intimate knowledge about how the food item being substituted tastes, smells, and the way it interacts with other food items, complimentary or otherwise. Also, some knowledge about the substitute is required. The reason for this is so that you will be able to select the best alternative that will give you similar if not equal satisfaction as what is being substituted.

Asafoetida is a favored spice used to prepare a considerable number of Indian dishes in particular, and Asian dishes in general. Hardly will you come across any traditional and indigenous Asian dish that has not been flavored with a dash of asafoetida or any of its substitutes. The substitutes in question will be adequately established later on in the chapter, but firstly, let us examine some of the reasons why asafoetida may be used as a substitute or may be substituted by other spices or food ingredients.

- Religious reasons
- Cultural reasons
- Allergy reasons

- Scarcity reasons
- Personal preference

Religious Reasons

In this instance, it is a two-sided coin. For the Hindus, the Buddhists, and the Jains who are not allowed to take garlic and onion during their religious rights, they use asafoetida instead to spice their food. On the other side of the coin, garlic and onion may be used in place of asafoetida.

Cultural Reasons

This has to do with customs and traditions that may have been passed down and may have been in existence for centuries. For instance, Jain ascetics are strict vegetarians. They also boycott any underground vegetables like onions, potatoes, garlic, etc. Therefore, asafoetida is used as a substitute in the cooking to give that coveted garlic and onion flavors to the food.

Allergy Reasons

Some people are allergic to certain spices, which means it must not be used to prepare their meals. If not, there will be dire consequences. Most people who are allergic to garlic also negatively react to leeks, chives, onions, and shallots. In which case, asafoetida comes to the rescue.

Scarcity Reasons

In parts of the world where asafoetida is not usually used, it might not be readily available and easy to get. In this case, substitutes are used instead.

Personal Preference

Asafoetida's natural foul smell might be a reason why some people prefer not to use it or even have anything to do with it at all. This applies to locust beans and any other unpleasantly smelling plant. In this case, the substitutes of it are used instead.

Asafoetida is not all about the flavor; it is perfect for medical purposes, especially for digestion; thus, people use it for its flavor and its health benefits. Therefore, if you are going to substitute it in your cooking, you have to try as much as possible to combine the choice substitutes with other supplementary ingredients like ginger, cumin powder, and fennel to achieve a similar effect health-wise, as if they had taken asafoetida instead.

The following are the substitutes of asafoetida and how they should be used to get favorably maximum results. Note that not all the substitutes are a perfect fit. Some are not so good for the purpose while some are better.

The substitutes;

- Garlic
- Onion
- Leeks

- Shallots
- Chives

Some of the substitutes listed above can be used relatively alone (e.g., garlic cloves) while some have to be used in conjunction with other substitutes to get the same effect (e.g., leeks and garlic, shallots and garlic, etc.)

Garlic; the different forms of garlic can be used as substitutes of asafoetida in the event of unavailability. However, the quantities and manner in which they are used vary.

- Garlic cloves; ½ teaspoon of asafoetida powder is equivalent to two finely sliced garlic cloves fricasseed in vegetable oil or ghee (highly prevalently used in Indian dishes). The quantity used may be adjusted based on your preference.
- Garlic powder; the substitute works wonders in situations whereby asafoetida is not the main spicing ingredient in the food. ½ teaspoon of garlic powder substitutes for ¼ of a teaspoon of asafoetida powder.
- Garlic flakes; one garlic clove = ½ teaspoon of garlic flakes. Therefore, a teaspoon of garlic flakes substitutes every ½ a teaspoon of asafoetida.

Onion; onion also substitutes asafoetida in different forms.

- Onion powder; onion powder, just like garlic powder, gives a low concentration of flavor; therefore, it should be used in situations that need asafoetida to be used very sparingly. For every ¼ teaspoon of asafoetida, ½ teaspoon of onion is required to substitute.
- Onion paste; this is made from blending freshly boiled onion into a paste. However, it is used with garlic for the best effect.

Onion and garlic; the combination here is applicable for finely sliced onion and garlic and onion and garlic powder. Combining these two substitutes gives a much better asafoetida flavor compared to using them alone. For every ¼ teaspoon of asafoetida powder, ¼ teaspoon of onion powder mixed with ¼ teaspoon of garlic powder would do the trick.

For the sliced variety, every ½ teaspoon of asafoetida powder, 1/3 cup of finely sliced yellow onion plus one finely sliced garlic clove fricasseed in vegetable oil or ghee is needed to substitute.

Sliced Leek and garlic; this combination gives one of the most potent substitutes of asafoetida. They could be blended together for a blander effect, or they could be fricasseed in oil or ghee. For every ½ teaspoon of asafoetida, combine 1/3 cup of finely sliced leek (naturally has a mild oniony flavor) and one finely sliced garlic clove.

Sliced shallots and garlic; a lot of people might opt for this combination because shallots give off a really lovely scent especially when fricasseed in oil. Shallots also have an oniony flavor albeit really mild. Combine 1/3 cup of finely sliced shallots and one finely sliced garlic clove for every ½ teaspoon of asafoetida.

Chives and Garlic; chives are of Chinese origin. They can be used as substitutes for garlic and onion. Therefore, combining them will deliver a very garlic-like or onion-like flavor to your dish as the case may be.

Chapter 4: How to Store Asafoetida

A lot has been said about the benefits of asafetida, but there are still more things you need to know; things like how to store and preserve the asafetida. To talk about storing it, we have to talk about extracting it and the forms in which it is available.

In the first chapter, the different forms in which you can get asafoetida were outlined. But how can you get them into those forms? Either you can cultivate the asafoetida plant, then harvest the resin gum yourself or you can go to the stores where they sell it - spice stores - and purchase it off the rack. These days, you could even buy it from stores online.

Actually, the cultivation option is stretching it a bit. The easiest way to get them is at a village market or farm market. In these markets, you can either get asafoetida in the unadulterated dried block form or in the unadulterated powdered form or granule form.

In the superstores, spice shops, and online stores, most of the asafoetidas sold are the adulterated ones. In other words, the raw asafoetida in block forms would have been ground into powder form and mixed with other ingredients especially wheat flour, rice flour, and Turmeric powder. They are then packaged in small airtight jars. The storage mechanism used from the stores might not be enough to keep the offensive smell of the spice in the jar. Therefore, you will need to take some storage measures.

Why Should You Take Storage Measures?

It is important to take storage measures to;

- Preserve the integrity (flavor, taste) of your spice, so it doesn't get contaminated.
- Inhibit the strong odor of asafoetida within the container it's kept in, so it doesn't contaminate other spices or the whole house at large.
- Make it easily assessable when it is needed.

Good storage practices

The importance of taking storage measures has been established. Now you need to know about how to take those measures properly. You need to imbibe good and efficient storage practices to keep your asafoetida fresh, flavorsome and readily available when you need it.

- Try as much as possible to purchase asafoetida that has not been crushed or adulterated, so that it is when you need some you grind it for use. The reason for this is that in the block form, it will last until you have exhausted it. However, in the spirit of being realistic, most people opt for convenience and, therefore, prefer to purchase the already ground and processed variety. Notwithstanding, if properly stored, it can also last for up to a year.
- So that your powdered asafoetida can last for the postulated one year or even more, it has to be kept in a cool and dry place where it will not be touched by air, water, and sunlight as these elements could degrade its potency and quality.

- A way to protect it from the elements is to be certain it is secured in an airtight container, preferably a glass container or a metal container (e.g., the Altoids tin of the old times). Keeping it in an airtight container/jar ensures that the smell does not seep out because it is strong enough to contaminate other spices or food items in close quarters, or even in the whole kitchen or pantry.
  For further fortification of the jar to make sure the smell does not escape, you can use rubber stoppers for the glass jars, or cover the opening of your chosen container with a small piece of polythene nylon before screwing the cover onto the container; this may seem strange to you, but it also helps to keep the smell in.
- Do not buy too much at a time. For powdered asafoetida, it is best to buy in quantities you are confident you will be able to exhaust. Resist the temptation of on-sale prices!
- Avoid keeping the asafoetida jars in the fridge or freezer. You can keep it in a cool place without putting it in the freezer. Keeping it at room temperature is ideal. The reason for the warning against keeping it in the freezer is because doing so will cause the spice to crystallize, and the process of thawing it every time you want to use it will allow humidity to contaminate it. The ideal place to store it is on the top shelves in your kitchen or pantry or any other elevated place.
- Label the asafoetida jar or container, so it is not mistaken for other spices in your spice collection, especially if you have other spices of similar colors. The funny thing here is that if you are not able to restrict asafoetida's distinctive smell to within the jar then mixing things up will not be a problem for you.

- Lastly, once you begin to notice that the spice has lost its distinctive smell or the potency of the smell has significantly reduced, then it is time to get rid of it. If you fail to do so and continue to use it, be ready for significant degradation of the flavor in your cooking.

Chapter 5: How to Cook and Recipes

Once the asafoetida is stored properly in your kitchen, you can then begin to use it to make as many delicacies as you like; there are a plethora of dishes you can make with asafetida. In some countries, it is a vital ingredient in some dishes such that without it, the food lacks the indigenous taste or the distinctive taste and flavor peculiar to it. For instance, in Iran asafoetida is vital in the making of meatballs, in Afghanistan asafoetida is used for cooking dried meat, in India appetizers, vegetables, pickles, and meat curries, among others, would not taste right without the use of asafoetida or at least its substitutes to flavor them.

There are various methods in which asafoetida is used to make food. Note that the block form of asafoetida cannot be used for cooking purposes unless it is crushed into powder or boiled in hot oil or water so that the oil and water extract is then used for cooking.

The following points outline how asafoetida is used for cooking with some tips here and there on how to maximize it.

- The raw block form of asafoetida is crushed, and the granular pieces are then blended with water to form a paste. This raw asafoetida paste is then introduced at the initial stage of cooking so that there is enough time for it to uniformly penetrate every corner of the food before it is done. This is necessary to achieve a balanced flavoring of the food.
- The paste or powdered asafoetida (especially the already adulterated ones) can also be stir-fried in hot oil

or ghee for few seconds before it is added to other ingredients or before other ingredients are added to it as the case may be. This method requires some caution as asafoetida can get easily burnt, especially if left to roast or fry for some time, even as short as thirty seconds.

Furthermore, this method of using asafoetida in your cooking requires you to add the stir-fried ingredient when the cooking is close to done, so the flavor does not mellow out. Therefore, use this method to cook foods that are ready within a short period. The reason for this is that the longer asafoetida is allowed to cook, the more its flavor deteriorates until it disappears altogether.

- Another method is to marinate your vegetables, meat, fish, chicken, etc., with the asafoetida paste or powder and all other spices; cumin, black pepper, ginger, etc. It is then put aside to marinate for at least two hours before it is fried or roasted.

- Lastly, you can boil asafoetida in water or add it to hot water to form a flavor induced water solution. This solution is then used as a cooking base for a lot of dishes; vegetable dishes, soups, meat, porridge, lentils, and any other dish you want to add it to.

Recipes that Include Asafoetida

There are thousands of recipes out there that incorporate asafoetida, particularly India and the subcontinent of India recipes. Writing all is not an option as there is no need to bore you with thousands of recipes you might not even need. Therefore, for illustration purposes, several recipes that reflect the methods of cooking with asafoetida explained above will be outlined.

Recipe One

Dish: chicken cooked in asafoetida sauce

Ingredients:

- 1 kg of chicken cubes
- 1 tablespoon (tbsp for short) of mustard oil
- 3 tbsp(s) of vegetable oil
- 1 teaspoon (tsp for short) of Ginger paste
- 2 bay leaves
- One cup of chopped fresh tomatoes
- 1 tsp of crushed chilly
- 1 tsp of cumin seeds
- 1 tsp of asafoetida powder
- 1 tsp of turmeric powder
- 1 tsp of cumin powder
- 1 tsp of chili powder
- ½ teaspoon of coriander powder
- Water (preferred quantity)
- Salt to taste

Directions:

- Fill a bowl with the chicken cubes; add the ginger paste, turmeric powder, coriander powder, chili powder, cumin powder, ¼ teaspoon of asafoetida powder, and the mustard oil. Mix thoroughly and set aside to marinate for at least three hours.
- Place a non-stick pot on the cooker and adjust heat to medium. Pour the vegetable oil and let it heat for a minute.
- Pour the cumin seeds and bay leaves into the hot oil and let it boil for thirty seconds, then add half a teaspoon of asafoetida. Let the mixture fry for another thirty seconds.
- Then add the pureed chicken and let it fricassee for about two minutes or until the chicken becomes uniformly golden yellow in color.
- Add the chopped tomatoes. Allow it to boil for about five minutes.
- Adjust the heat to low, add the crushed chili.
- If it is too thick, add water and allow boil until you can clearly differentiate the oil from the rest of the mixture.
- Put salt until the taste is satisfactory.
- Dish with boiled rice or bread.

The recipe above was used because it illustrates the use of asafoetida to marinate and stir fry in the cooking process.

Recipe Two

Dish: Rasam (a south Indian soup usually taken as an appetizer)

Ingredients:

- 3 sizable fresh tomatoes
- 5 curry leaves
- A handful of coriander leaves (chopped)
- ½ tsp of cumin seeds
- 1 tsp of ginger powder
- ½ tsp of mustard seed
- 1 tsp of peppercorns
- ½ tsp of ghee
- A pinch of asafoetida
- Water (2 cups)
- Salt to taste

Directions:

- Get a bowl with lukewarm water. Add 2 pinch of salt. Thoroughly rinse the fresh tomatoes in the solution to remove any contaminants.
- Pour 4 tsp of water into a grinder. Add the freshly washed tomatoes, ginger powder, cumin seeds, asafoetida, coriander leaves, peppercorns, and curry leaves
- Grind everything together to form a paste.
- Place a pan on the cooker and adjust the flame to medium heat. Pour the two cups of water into the pan. Add the paste. Cover the pan and allow the mixture to boil. Stir for a minute. Put off the flame and set aside for now.

- Place another pan on the flame (same medium heat flame). Add the ghee and the mustard seed. Allow mixture to fry for twenty seconds.
- Pour the fried mixture into the tomato paste mixture earlier set aside, and then add the curry leaves and green chili if you have.
- Put salt until you are satisfied with the taste.
- Fry the mixture until it crackles.
- You can serve with chutneys or papads or both.

In the recipe above, asafoetida was blended with other ingredients into a paste which is then boiled, thus, illustrating yet another way to use asafoetida for cooking.

Chapter 6: Where to Buy Asafoetida

If you cannot find it in your local street market, maybe because it is not cultural to have Asafoetida there, you can find it in Amazon where I buy all my herbs and supplements.

Just search for "Asafoetida" in Amazon and pick the best reviewed products.

Below I give you a few recommendations with my affiliate Amazon links. They won't cost you anything more, but the commission does help to fill my coffee fund and keep me writing – so thanks if you do ;)

Asafoedita Yellow 100g (Hing)

QiVeda Asafoetida Powder (Hing) | USDA Organic | Grain & Gluten Free (3.53 oz.)

Food of the Gods" Asafetida Powder (Asafoetida) - 100% Organic & Natural

Asafoetida (Hing) Organic 2.8 OZ

Indiveda Whole Asafoetida (Heeng) - Strong Aroma

Conclusion

The Persians named asafoetida the 'food of the gods.' This title is a tribute to the curative capabilities and multitudes of health benefits it presents. The objective of this book is to reinforce the interest of those who already know about the wonderful spice/vegetable and to encourage those who may have heard about it but have not tried it to do so. Asafoetida has a magical way of transforming the flavor of any dish if applied in the right way, regardless of its unpleasant natural odor. The so-called discomfort from the smell pales in comparison to the multitudes of benefits it promises.

Apart from the adverse health issues that asafoetida causes when used in large quantities, there are also food dangers if it is not used sparingly. Just a pinch of it goes a long way in improving the flavor of your food. However, if you use too much of it, you might not like the results at all. The message here is that asafoetida has to be used as sparingly as possible for you to get the best out of it.

A parting word for my dear reader, eating food is not just all about the taste or the satisfaction you get from it, you should eat for the benefits it promises your body health-wise. Your body is like a machine, and the food ingested is the fuel that runs it; therefore, fuel it with the good stuff. If you have not been doing that, it is not too late, start with asafetida.

Thank you!

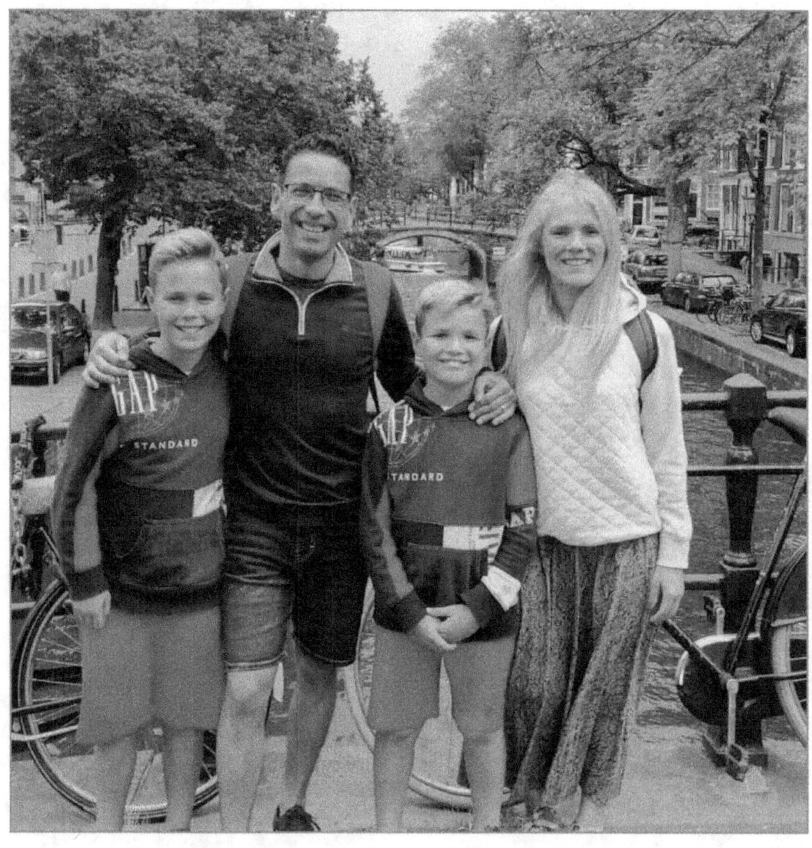

Hope you liked the book and please reread/study it!
Please leave a review in order to help me as an author and to improve and refine the content of this book.
Your review is very important. I will read it very carefully as it will be used as a tool to deliver better books! Many thanks in advance!
Please go to your account on Amazon or click on the link below.
[CLICK HERE TO LEAVE A REVIEW ON AMAZON!](#)
Thank you and good luck! Cheers!

Resources

https://draxe.com/nutrition/asafoetida/

https://www.naturalnews.com/2018-07-17-asafoetida-a-plant-used-in-traditional-folk-medicines-found-to-show-antitumor-effects-on-breast-cancer.html

https://www.netmeds.com/health-library/post/hing-medicinal-uses-therapeutic-benefits-for-gut-health-and-recipes

https://www.thekitchn.com/inside-the-spice-cabinet-asafoetida-or-asafetida-140001

http://saltandtamarind.com/asafoetida/
https://www.organicfacts.net/health-benefits/other/asafoetida.html

https://www.astrogle.com/ayurveda/ferula-asafoetida-medicinal-usage-side-effects-warnings.html

https://www.herbal-supplement-resource.com/asafetida-benefits.html

https://www.sharecare.com/health/herbal-supplements/what-are-warnings-for-asafoetida

https://draxe.com/nutrition/asafoetida/

https://www.naturalnews.com/2018-07-17-asafoetida-a-plant-used-in-traditional-folk-medicines-found-to-show-antitumor-effects-on-breast-cancer.html

https://www.greenmedinfo.com/substance/asafoetida

https://articles.mercola.com/sites/articles/archive/2020/01/13/asafoetida-benefits.aspx

https://www.netmeds.com/health-library/post/hing-medicinal-uses-therapeutic-benefits-for-gut-health-and-recipes

https://www.organicfacts.net/health-benefits/other/asafoetida.html

http://healthblog247.com/health-benefits-of-asafetida-or-hing/

https://holisticzine.com/asafoetida-benefits

https://food.ndtv.com/food-drinks/10-amazing-health-benefits-of-asafoetida-we-should-all-know-about-1825666

http://healthblog247.com/health-benefits-of-asafetida-or-hing/

https://ifood.tv/ingredients/356425-asafoetida-substitutes-top-asafetida-substitutes

https://tastessence.com/asafoetida-substitute

https://www.gourmetsleuth.com/ingredients/detail/asafoetida

https://www.greedygourmet.com/ingredients/asafoetida-substitutes/

https://oureverydaylife.com/substitutes-for-asafetida-powder-12554266.html

https://thespiceguide.com/whats-the-best-substitute-for-asafoetida/
https://nutrineat.com/how-to-cook-with-asafoetida

https://www.yummytummyaarthi.com/homemade-asafoetida-recipe-hing/

http://saltandtamarind.com/asafoetida/

https://www.gourmetsleuth.com/ingredients/detail/asafoetida

https://forums.egullet.org/topic/44163-phew-asafoetida-storage/

https://nutrineat.com/how-to-cook-with-asafoetida

https://www.netmeds.com/health-library/post/hing-medicinal-uses-therapeutic-benefits-for-gut-health-and-recipes

https://www.tarladalal.com/glossary-asafoetida-113i

https://www.seattletimes.com/life/food-drink/asafoetida-stinks-but-it-helps-the-cook/

https://www.bbc.co.uk/food/asafoetida

https://draxe.com/nutrition/asafoetida/